CW00520667

ALZHEIMER'S TIMELINE

A Layman's Study of Dementia in the Family

Brian Bailie

Copyright © 2011 Brian Bailie

All rights reserved.

ISBN: 9781456605544

dedicated to my sister-in-law, Janet

without whom this would have been a very different story

£1.00

CONTENTS

Introduction

I am just the son of a beautiful woman whose mind was stolen from her.

I'm not a doctor, I need a spell-checker to write *psychiatrist*. I have no medical education or experience. And there are *millions* of people just like me, who really don't understand half the information we're told by health professionals. So I want to just describe my experience of Alzheimer's disease in my family, in plain language, like it was, and how it is.

Over the past twelve years or so, Mum's mind has dissolved relentlessly, like sugar in warm water, and it has left her in a perpetual existence of total inability and total dependency.

Yes, this is a personal, frequently embarrassing and very emotional story for me to write. But I know that my mum would want her experience and suffering to be used to help and prepare others; to help you avoid the mistakes that I made; to speak to you in the honest words of a simple helpless layman.

The thing about hindsight is that it only makes you wiser if you're going to do something over again. I don't like to think about having to care for another loved one with dementia, but I'd like to think that my story *will* help others. So the sole reason for publishing this account of my mum's decline is the hope that *my* experience and *my* hindsight will help you: Help you to anticipate problems; Help you to plan care arrangements; Help you to realise the importance of legal and financial issues; and Help you to prepare practically and emotionally.

I've had to walk a delicate line: I have a younger sister, and an elder brother. Hilary was happy enough for me to make decisions and change things within reason, but because Paul is older than me, I really felt that he should have been more involved with the significant decisions, especially any decisions to do with moving money around, or spending it. But Paul had emigrated years ago, and so his involvement was limited to his opinion, and his approval or disapproval.

Trust is the key. Not that I *was* mistrusted, but the first decision I made about my involvement with Mum and Dad was that *everything* that I did must be totally transparent. Consequently, the only reason that I can catalogue Mum's decline so accurately is because I put everything in writing: every event, every decision, every incident, every diagnosis was written down and emailed to Paul as it happened. So this little book, and the accuracy of the timeline of Mum's decline into total dependency, is the direct result of my correspondence with my brother.

*To help me identify the clinical stages of my mum's Alzheimer's disease I'm using the **Seven-Stage Scale** developed by renowned Alzheimer's specialist, **Dr Barry Reisberg**. This is known as the **Global Deterioration Scale**. This scale is used by mental health professionals to categorise the phases of degeneration with Alzheimer's disease.*

STAGE ONE

No Cognitive Decline

No subjective complaints of memory deficit. No memory deficit evident on clinical interview.

Global Deterioration Scale © Barry Reisberg, MD

Well that's reassuring: we're all at least Stage 1 of dementia, like a ticking time bomb that may, or may not have a detonator. It isn't very helpful. Is this just some over-analytical chin-stroker trying to be clever; or *should* I be worried?

If I summarised Mum's character before she began to suffer from dementia, I would describe a very fun and child-like personality. Mum was out-going, loving, trusting, a little naïve perhaps, perpetually happy, and a little too selfless. She was also dippy, scatty, disorganised, untidy, through-other, and may have been described as happy-go-lucky. Everyone loved Mum, and Mum loved everyone. I don't think any of these characteristics can be identified as anything other than perfectly normal. However, I accept that most of these characteristics can *also* be identified as symptoms of something more sinister.

STAGE TWO

Very Mild Cognitive decline

Subjective complaints of memory deficit, most frequently in following areas:

> *(a) forgetting where one has placed familiar objects;*
>
> *(b) forgetting names one formerly knew well.*

No objective evidence of memory deficit on clinical interview. No objective deficits in employment or social situations. Appropriate concern with respect to symptomatology.

Global Deterioration Scale © Barry Reisberg, MD

But everyone does this (don't they?). I frequently forget the name of my dogs, (that's why I've trained them to come to my whistle). And of course I know the names of my own children, but occasionally, mid-sentence, I might refer to them with another familiar name. It's frustrating for me, and it's annoying for my child; but is this dementia? Of course it isn't, it's just normal. Everyone does it.

You mean to tell me that you've never gone to get something, walked into a room to get it, and stood there like an eejit trying to remember why you're there and what you're looking for? We all do stuff like this. It's called being relaxed; your brain is on stand-by, we're just mentally freewheeling (aren't we?). I think that what the Global Deterioration Scale wants to emphasise is that this kind of forgetfulness is a symptom of Stage 2, however it's also a symptom of being a relaxed, perfectly healthy human being.

To put this into the context of my mum's early symptoms, no one noticed anything, because as I've already described her, she had always been dippy, scatty, and disorganised. And with Dad beginning to suffer from ill health, Mum was bound to be worried, I never thought twice about her being a little more disorganised or more forgetful than usual.

STAGE THREE

Mild Cognitive Decline (Mild Cognitive Impairment)

Earliest clear-cut deficits.

Manifestations in more than one of the following areas:

(a) patient may have gotten lost when traveling to an unfamiliar location;

(b) co-workers become aware of patient's relatively poor performance;

(c) word and name finding deficit becomes evident to intimates;

(d) patient may read a passage or a book and retain relatively little material;

(e) patient may demonstrate decreased facility in remembering names upon introduction to new people;

(f) patient may have lost or misplaced an object of value;

(g) concentration deficit may be evident on clinical testing. Objective evidence of memory deficit obtained only with an intensive interview. Decreased performance in demanding employment and social settings. Denial begins to become manifest in patient. Mild to moderate anxiety accompanies symptoms.

Global Deterioration Scale © Barry Reisberg, MD

Brian Bailie

10

STAGE 3 TIMELINE: **October 2000 – July 2002**

Behaviour timeline:

* Noticing that Mum was becoming unusually forgetful.
* Professionals showing concern for the consequences of Mum's scattiness.
* Friends and family showing concern for Mum's confusion.
* Frustration at my inability to reason with Mum.
* Mum's resentment of the introduction of assistance.
* Mum's continual denial of any problem with her memory.
* Questioning if Mum's condition *is* dementia, or if it *could* be just stress-related.
* Mum's occasional ability to demonstrate lucidity to disguise her inner confusion.
* Mum's neglect of her own personal hygiene.

Event timeline:

* The eventual realisation that Mum needed help and support.
* Difficulty and reluctance to interfere with Mum's established position within the family.
* My difficulty making the transition from child of a parent, to decision-maker of the parent.
* Disagreements between siblings about what to do and how to handle Mum's condition.
* Family feelings of frustration and helplessness.
* Diplomatic introduction of assistance for Mum to aid her care of Dad.
* Taking control of Mum and Dad's finances.
* Taking control of Dad's care away from Mum.

You see, I knew Mum was making mistakes and forgetting things, and the house was a mess. But she was caring for Dad, who was diabetic and had already suffered a few mini-strokes, and he was becoming more and more dependent and demanding on Mum. So *naturally* Mum was stressed, and stressed people get confused and forget things.

Things came to a head on **2nd October 2000**. My sister, Hilary, had arranged to take Mum out for coffee and window-shopping; so Mum had arranged to collect Dad's sister so that she could sit with Dad and keep him company while they were out. But when Hilary arrived, Mum was still away collecting Dad's sister, and the nurse was leaving the house saying that Dad had decided to stay in bed today.

Hilary brought the nurse back into the house, and together they turfed Dad out of his lazy bed, got him dressed and seated in his grumpy chair in the lounge, ready for his sister. But when Mum returned, Hilary realised that coffee and window-shopping wasn't going to happen that day. Dad's sister drifted into the room like a frozen knitwear model, staring into the middle distance and smiling like an idiot. Mum had two dosey old trouts to care for now. So, very frustrated, Hilary excused herself and drove down the peninsula to visit me at my little workshop.

That morning's events were the wake-up call that made us realise that Mum needed help caring for Dad, whether she wanted it or not, whether she continued to insist that she was *fine*, or not. Mum was becoming exhausted with stress, and if things continued the way they were going, Dad would probably outlive her.

I spent days on the phone with social services, trying to arrange day-care for Dad; somewhere that he would be bathed, entertained, and fed, and returned after a few hours respite for Mum. But there were only fifty-five daycare places available for the whole of the North Down area (which has a population exceeding 80,000), and there was a long, long waiting-list; and even if Dad *was* accepted for day-care, it would only be for one afternoon each week.

So I reckoned that if I couldn't get Dad out of the house for respite, I'd arrange to get Mum out. By **10th October 2000** I had secured the professional services of a reputable day-care service. By 11th October, Mum had objected to the cost, and I had foolishly allowed her to persuade me to rearrange a similar service with a much cheaper organisation (£2 cheaper, by the hour). Anyhow, it was finally arranged that a carer would come and sit with Dad between 10am and 2pm, two days each week.

Hooray, Mum could go out now. The carer could make Dad's lunch, toilet him, light the fire, chat with Dad, watch TV with him, tidy up a little; and Mum had a little regular freedom. That was the idea. However I was still a little uneasy about the quality of this care package. I had originally arranged this service with a very reputable care agency; and Mum had asked me to rearrange it with this other one that operated from an unlisted phone number answered by the owner's mother. But what could go wrong?

I'd received a very humiliating phone call from the owner of the first (reputable) care agency. The owner explained to me that the person I now had looking after my Dad used to work for her agency – as the cleaner, but she had to fire her because she was so unreliable. (Well she seemed to be a very enterprising unreliable cleaner.) You get what you pay for, I guess, and to appease Mum, I was stuck with this care package, such as it was.

On the **20th November 2000** Mum left for a holiday with her best friend: off to visit my brother Paul in Bermuda for a week. This wasn't easy to organise. Mum *really* didn't want to go; she didn't want to leave Dad. But it seemed perfect: travelling with her best friend, staying with her son on a beautiful island, off-season relaxation; it was a perfect way to wind down, (wouldn't you think?).

I'd secured a room for Dad at a good care home while Mum was away; yet, despite Dad getting off to a great start, after a couple of days I received an unfriendly phone call from the head keeper who stated that Dad was too much for them to handle, and that he needed to be moved to a nursing home – immediately. Dad was being expelled.

Dad's expulsion was embarrassing for me, and should've been humiliating for Dad, but he didn't seem to care anymore. He was still in bed in his tiny room when I arrived alone to remove him. His room stank. He resisted any attempts to move him, so that it became a physical struggle between the two of us. I could've cried at the pathetic state of my dad, but a small crowd had gathered to watch from the corridor, and among those staring aghast were two of his oldest and dearest friends.

I propped Dad up in the wheelchair, held my head high in defiance of the horrified glares I was receiving, and wheeled Dad from the building knowing that our voyeurs were whispering, "D'you know who that old man used to be....?"

I was very unhappy with the first nursing home I took him to. When I discovered him neglected the next day, sitting in front of the telly, sitting in his own shit, I abducted him there and then and took him to another nursing home over in Comber. That wasn't ideal either, but Dad was more content, and I was less concerned.

One thing I now realised for certain: no way should Mum be caring for Dad alone. If a care home couldn't care for him, if he needed nursing care, then Mum wasn't able for this. No wonder she was going daft.

I hear you: *Why did it take this incident to make me realise that my own mum needed more help than she was receiving?* It's not that simple. And she *was* receiving assistance: a nurse came to help get Dad out of bed and dressed in the morning, and another came in the evening to help him back to bed. But in-between these visits, Mum was the sole carer. And she forcefully rejected any suggestion that Dad be cared for in any other way, or by any other person.

D'you know what I mean? I'm not making excuses: Mum bluntly refused to accept the fact that she couldn't care properly for Dad.

- With hindsight, this *was* a symptom of dementia.
- With hindsight, Mum was probably killing Dad with her best intentions.

While Mum was visiting Paul I spoke with her doctor.

This is another significant stepping-stone in the role-reversal of parent and child. I call it *interfering*, because it feels everything like interfering. It's a difficult line to cross; but for the sake of my dad, I really didn't have an option.

Like me, Mum's doctor wasn't convinced that Mum's confusion was anything more than stress-related; but a close family friend whose wife had recently died with Alzheimer's disease, persuaded me that dementia was a <u>real</u> possibility, so I reluctantly requested that a psychiatric examination be arranged for Mum's return from holiday, (I would tell her that it was just to test for stress, not dementia).

17

Mum returned from her holiday in Bermuda, and returned to her routine of intensive care for Dad. And soon any benefits that she may have enjoyed from her holiday were wasted, (or forgotten).

The casual day-carer was back again for two days each week; but this benefit took a swift nose-dive when Mum delightedly informed me that the carer was pregnant (Mum and Dad never had kids of their own ((we three are adopted)) and Mum always got very excited when someone else announced that they were expecting a baby). The inevitable happened quicker than I'd expected. I called one morning to find Dad and his carer sitting watching telly in front of a lovely fire, while Mum was preparing a large roast chicken dinner for them all. Yes, Mum was now caring for the carer too.

By **24th December 2000** I'd had enough, *again*.

I was constantly receiving phone calls from friends and relations telling me how worried they were for Mum, and saying how awful it is to see her like that (*these phone calls were just the worst, and made me feel like such a failure*). Mum's friends and family were asking when is something going to be done to help her; and what am I doing about it? But I couldn't do anything, I couldn't do a bloody thing because every time I tried to help Mum she un-helped herself and made things ten times worse: caring for Dad's carer; having a totally spoilt and undisciplined dirty dog rule the house; forgetting to pay bills, or lodge cheques; not replacing her home-help (who had left because of ill-health) in case she offended her,......... and her house looked like an earthquake in a charity shop.

I was boiling with frustration when I visited Mum on Christmas Eve.

I told her that I loved her. I told her that I knew that I was interfering with her life. I told her that I was interfering with her life *because* I loved her, and that I was only trying to help her; but I wasn't going to be pussy-footing around her anymore. If I saw something that needed done, I'd do it whether she liked it or not. I told her that she had to realise that she needed help. I made her cry. And she agreed that she needed help, and that I should continue to *interfere*.

Hilary and I had fallen out that Christmas. I'd said to Mum that having Hilary's kids to stay over only made a confused situation worse; and Mum had told Hilary that I had said that her kids were not allowed to visit at all. We were both feeling very tense and worried about Mum and Dad, and on **New Year's Day 2001** I'd driven to Bangor to visit Hilary and put things right, and call with Mum and Dad.

This wasn't *just* a result of a misunderstanding, or a misinterpreted message. Hilary and I are naturally very close, but the anxiety and heightened tension caused by seeing our mum in confused distress caring for our dying dad, and not knowing what to do or how to offer practical help, had made us both very tetchy and touchy (because we both felt we were failing our parents). We sorted things out between us; we'd achieve nothing disunited.

A perfect metaphor met me when I arrived at Mum's driveway. I'd spent the previous afternoon in foul winter weather scraping back the snow and ice from Mum's path, and hauling buckets of sand off the beach to spread about so that it was safe for her to walk outside. But the wind had shifted in the night, the ice and snow had melted, and I was left with a sandy mess to start clearing up. One step forward, two steps back; the more I tried to help, the bigger the mess I had to deal with. It summed it all up, and I was resigned to more grief even before I reached the front door.

Inside was the usual organised pandemonium, but today there was a horrific stink, like a Chinese public toilet. Dad's bottom had exploded, again.

A few months earlier I had taken everything out of the dining room and bunged it all upstairs so that I could bring Mum and Dad's bedroom downstairs so that Dad didn't need to negotiate the stairs twice a day. This seemed like a good idea, until his bottom occasionally exploded.

The problem (identified with the crystal clarity of hindsight) was that Mum was treating Dad for constipation, *and* treating him for constipation, *and then* treating him for constipation. She had no idea how many times she had administered a laxative, but if Dad's bottom could speak we might have a good idea; if Dad's bottom could speak it might have whimpered, "Help me" because it later turned out that Mum was treating him (and over-treating him) for constipation, and then treating him (and over-treating him) for diarrhoea, so that his bowels were being medicated from one extreme to the other in a cycle of advanced geological proportions.

Dad's morning and evening nurses got in touch with me. They were very concerned about Dad's care. They were

21

sure that Mum was over- and under-dosing him with whatever she had available, and Mum wasn't keeping any records and couldn't remember when Dad was last given medicine, or what that medicine might have been.

It turned out that Mum was also forgetting to feed Dad some mealtimes (which as you know is dangerous for a diabetic), or feeding him twice in succession, not remembering if she had or hadn't. And Dad was too miserably *out of it* to complain.

So I asked, and received, a third daily nursing visit, this one in the mid-afternoon.

I called with Mum to explain. And I also told Mum that the nurses would be giving Dad his medicine, so it was one less thing for her to have to think about. This was an imposition, and she told me so. Mum said that she "Wasn't away with the fairies just yet" (says I, that'll be a relief for the fairies.)

Among a pile of junk and papers I noticed a letter outlined in red. It was from Readers Digest, stating that they still hadn't received the outstanding £17.50 and that the matter was now in the hands of their debt-collectors. My eyes scanned the room for more letters, and sure enough I discovered another from Sun Life Assurance........., if I could find important letters like these without trying, what other letters were lurking about the house?

I sat with Dad on the evening of **3rd January 2001** while Mum went out with a friend. He was great. I made supper, we watched some telly, we made three uneventful but productive visits to the toilet, and I gave him a clean close shave. He was in good humour; and then Mum returned and it was all fuss-fuss-fuss, and Dad mentally withdrew. This wasn't how it should be. My dad was unhappy.

I *was* trying to help.

Mum didn't want Dad taking any respite at the nursing home because it cost so much, and said that she was perfectly capable of caring for him herself; the day-carer was reduced to one afternoon each week, *"because she's pregnant dear"* and should be at home; and the convene was a complete waste of time. I'd asked the nurses to fit Dad with a convene so that he could wee where he sat, and it saves repeated visits to the toilet for a dribble-piddle. But Mum kept a close eye on this convene thing, and as soon as she noticed any amount of wee in it, off they went to the loo. So what's the point? What was the *bloody* point?

The obvious solution now would've been to live with Mum. That's the ideal scenario: move in, oversee everything, be there for moral support, sort the mail, pay the bills on time, keep Dad happy, and help to keep Mum sane. But life's not like that.

My self-employment had been reduced to about two days actual work each week because of my commitment to Mum and Dad; I had a family to provide for; and I lived about forty minutes away, so even a ten minute visit to Mum was a big chunk out of my day.

Could I have closed my business, and moved my family to live with Mum and Dad? Nothing's impossible. It was a great location, walking distance to the town, and right on the shore; but I couldn't commit myself to a plan. I couldn't ask my Claire to live with my disorganised mum and dependant dad in this house of pandemonium. And even if we did move in, what happens when Dad dies and if Mum needs to go into care? My family would be homeless. I couldn't move in, even if I should have.

Things continued until **March 2001**, when Mum told me that Dad hadn't had a bowel movement for about a month, but not to worry because she'd been dosing him up on laxatives for the past few days,...... *Great Balls of Fire: my dad was an unexploded bomb on a Zimmer Frame.*

On 7th **March** poor Dad's bottom finally erupted, everywhere, and the house stank again.

I spoke with Mum's best friend, and it was arranged that they take a short break to the Mournes and stay at a nice hotel for the weekend, and I would arrange for Dad to get a bed in a nursing home: respite for both.

I don't think Mum's forgetfulness appeared to get worse during these months, but she was still very forgetful. She forgot to take any food or drink on a picnic; she forgot that she already had a birthday present for my son, and gave him money too, and then apologised for not bringing a card after she had just given him one. And she refused to believe that Dad was as weak and ill as he clearly was. But none of this was shocking forgetfulness, and we still convinced ourselves that it couldn't be dementia – Mum was too young. She was just 69 years old.

Mum still took Dad out places, pulling him along by his Zimmer Frame. She was in denial that Dad was deteriorat-

ing, and she kept talking about his condition as if she was waiting for him to get better.

Poor Dad. Mum forgot to button his trousers in a res-
taurant toilet, and when they started walking down High
Street, Dad's trousers dropped to his ankles. And also, one
early evening Mum and Dad visited us so she could go to my
kids' school play while I sat with Dad. Claire and I were looking after twin babies at that time, and I'd just popped upstairs
to check on them, but when I returned Dad was gone. I discovered him outside lying on the path with his trousers down,
shit everywhere. He'd needed the toilet, and had tried to get
outside to avoid a mess in the house. He was pathetic. This
smelly old man had been such a well-respected gentleman:
businessman, Alderman, J.P., chairman of more than a dozen
public committees; and he was lying outside distressed, un-
dressed, and moaning like a drunk. I felt totally worthless as a
son. The shit was everywhere and I had to cut his clothes off
him before bringing him inside to wash. How could Mum say
that she was coping with Dad when I couldn't even leave for
him alone for three minutes?

Mum still hadn't been referred for psychiatric examination.

No, that's not correct. What I should say is that a mental health expert still hadn't examined Mum. She *had* been referred, but the appointment letter had been sent to *Mum*, and naturally enough she had lost it.

Mum had an appointment with her doctor for 10:30 on **24th May 2001.**

I phoned and spoke to the doctor at 10:25 and offloaded as much background information as I could remember about Mum and her forgetful, disorganised condition, and how it was affecting Dad. The doctor was very sympathetic and understanding.

I phoned Mum when she returned from the appointment to ask how she got on. She said she thought the doctor wasn't much good, "He didn't even take my blood pressure."

The doctor immediately made another appointment for Mum with the Mental Health Clinic, for 7th June.

Mum phoned to cancel this mental health appointment, saying that she would be away that day, rambling at Por-

27

trush. The clinic gave her another appointment date – but she couldn't remember where she wrote it down.

Mum didn't go to Portrush. She said that Dad wouldn't have enjoyed it anyway. But I already knew the real reason. Dad had been to his weekly visit to the day-care centre, and his bottom exploded. He had been stripped, washed, wrapped in blankets, and delivered home again in a hurry.

Dad was in a bad state. As I'd arranged in January, the nurses were administering Dad's insulin, however the nurses strongly suspected that Mum was also injecting Dad with insulin. The nurses were very frustrated and very worried for Dad's quality of life, (previously, as Chairman of the Health Committee, Dad had presented many of these nurses with their qualification certificates, now they were watching him being cared to death).

I phoned the Mental Health Clinic and pleaded for an early appointment. 11th July, *if* the doctor doesn't take a holiday.

In the meantime I arranged for Dad to go for emergency respite care in a nursing home, and for Mum to go for a long weekend to Kildare with her best friend.

Dad was very weak now; weak and frequently confused, and he sometimes struck out at the nurses. The doctor had prescribed diazepam to keep him settled.

Mum returned from Kildare and phoned me, looking for Dad. I asked her how she enjoyed her holiday: "What holiday, dear?"

"Your long weekend in Kildare. You stayed in a bed & breakfast over a pub."

"No dear, I don't think so."

Okay so, Mum stayed the weekend in a room above a pub in rural Ireland, and she doesn't remember it. (Those Irish pubs must be so quiet at the weekends.)

Hilary had quite a serious traffic collision at the end of June. She was T-boned at a busy junction, and both cars were wrecked. Mum asked Hilary where her car was, and Hilary said it had been destroyed in a car-crash. Mum just laughed and said, "Och, Hilary. You're awful."

Mum's social worker had notified Social Services about her concerns. They sent a team of their people to assess her, (no one knew about this until after they'd been). They interviewed Mum, and sent their report to Mum's social worker.

Their report stated that they were originally convinced that they'd gone to the wrong house because everything was fine, Mum was great and showed no signs of stress; and Dad appeared to be well cared for............. I felt like a complete tit. The nurses were dumbfounded, and the social worker was speechless, ... It just shows you how well Mum could disguise her confusion (or how inexperienced the assessment team was).

11ᵗʰ July 2001 I arrived to collect Mum for her appointment, (THE appointment).

I explained that we had a routine appointment to go to, and without a problem off we merrily went. Mum was relaxed and fine about the whole thing, until we entered the hospital car park.

I scanned the surrounding buildings searching for directions, mumbling, "Where *is* the building?" And then my heart sank to my boots. There it was in front of me: the one with the huge sign over the door that read, MENTAL HEALTH CLINIC.

Mum began to panic. I began to panic. I reassured her that we were just going in to have a chat about her stress, and how they may be able to help her. We held hands like a nervous child and parent on the first day of school (except that I was the parent, and Mum was the child).

They didn't keep us waiting too long, *but it seemed like a very long time*. Mum became more and more apprehensive and fidgety, up and down from her seat and me after her, until she was finally called.

Again I held her by the hand and we entered a dreary little room decorated unwelcoming grey, with a window that faced out towards a brick wall. It was like a prison cell, and I knew that Mum felt trapped.

The psychiatrist was friendly enough, perhaps a little too patronising and sweet. She opened her papers and started to engage with Mum. I'm so glad I was with her. I was so glad I was able to joke and make little of the questions that Mum couldn't answer. Really, the horrible unfriendly room, the questioning, the deliberate noting of Mum's answers: it was all very intimidating, so much so that if it had been me being questioned, I'm sure that I'd have fluffed a few answers.

We would hear the results of this first interview in a week or so, but I already knew that Mum's forgetfulness wasn't normal, and probably wasn't *just* caused by the stress of caring for her dying husband.

The psychiatrist's report stated that there was strong likelihood that Mum had Alzheimer's disease, and they wanted a blood test to confirm the diagnosis. This changed things. This changed things a lot. This changed any plans for Mum's future, and the family's involvement, *if* this diagnosis was correct.

But my priority right now was focused on Dad and his future (how ever long that might be). Dad was going to need proper nursing care, and this wasn't going to be cheap.

In **August 2001** I began to I search for the deeds of the house. I needed to know whether their house was in Dad's name, or Dad and Mum jointly, because Mum could be made homeless if Dad's nursing fees had to be paid from his assets. The deeds were not to be found at their house, nor in their deed box, nor with his solicitor; so I asked the bank if they still held the deeds, but they said that they didn't have them either. They were lost.

What I *did* find on my hunt through Mum's house were un-presented cheques, and letters from various institutions enquiring about cheques they'd sent to Dad that had never been presented. Several thousand pounds had been mislaid in these missing cheques.

- I wrote a letter for Mum to sign to each of the various financial institutions and asked them to cancel any un-presented cheques, and to either re-issue them or to make payment directly into Dad's bank account.
- I asked Mum to sign a mandate for the bank to permit me access to and authority over their bank accounts.
- I instructed Dad's solicitor to prepare the documentation we needed to appoint Hilary and me joint Power of Attorney over Mum.

The other thing I did was remove weeks of growth from Dad's chin. Dad had never worn facial hair, he always kept himself clean-shaven, even on holiday; but he was beginning to look like Santa's daddy.

A new nursing care package took effect for Dad. The nurses did everything, and Mum was forced to take a backseat. A proper hospital bed arrived for Dad, and this required more shifting of stuff about their house to make room, and I set up a single bed for Mum beside his.

Their house was indescribably messy and cluttered and disorganised. But it was impossible to do anything productive about it all because Mum didn't want anything disturbed. But I kept finding important documents and more un-presented cheques lying about, which meant that if any tidy-up was to take place, every single piece of paper would have to be examined, every pile of magazines, newspapers and junk mail checked, page-by-page. And Hilary and I knew from attempting to tidy up before, that as soon as you clear one space, almost simultaneously Mum just comes along and messes it up with more stuff. It was depressing, and despite everything I did, and all the time I'd taken off work to try to help, I felt it was all totally wasted, a complete waste of my time and effort and emotional energy. What made it worse was Mum's silly attitude to it all, like these cheques didn't matter, like I don't need to work to make money, like it's just a little game; and everything can be made better with a hug and a kiss. <u>It can't.</u>

Mum would drive into town for a message, and lose her car in the car park and have to walk home; she was cycling along to the local shops, and walking home having forgotten all about her bicycle; she was going shopping without money, and writing cheques for pennies; she was agreeing to buy ridiculously unsuitable things from door-to-door salesmen (because they were so nice to her),.....

It was only a matter of time before Mum would do something that could result in damage or injury to another person, or herself. As far as I could see, the only obvious solution was for either Hilary or I to move in to live with Mum, (*and then we could all go mad together*).

By the middle of **September 2001** Dad had been admitted to hospital. Mum spent every day with him, trying to nurse and feed him. I think Dad would've been happier without Mum's relentless attention at this point, but she demanded to be there, constantly. She only went home in the evening because her dog needed fed (and to clear up the wee and pooh that the dog had had to make while it had been locked in the house all day).

35

Once Dad's condition had been stabilised he was brought back home in late September. He had a complete care package that was supposed to eliminate Mum from his care, but I'm sure she continued to have a negative affect on his condition.

Mum was due an appointment for her second assessment at the Mental Health Clinic, but after Hilary described a particularly difficult shopping expedition with Mum I phoned the clinic and managed to bring this appointment forward to 4th October 2001.

I sat in with Mum again. The same dreary, cell-like interrogation room. The same memory questions......., *what day is it; what month is it; who is the Prime Minister,........?* And Mum scored the same results as her first examination.

12th October 2001 Dad was admitted to hospital again. I phoned Mum to find out why. She didn't know (or didn't remember); in fact Mum thought that I'd arranged Dad's hospitalisation, and she asked me the same question. It was all a big laugh to Mum; she didn't seem to be worried in the slightest.

Hilary phoned me. She'd spoken with the hospital. Dad had been taken into hospital because his swallow was poor, and he was excessively lethargic. Within a couple of days Dad was rehydrated, fresh faced again, and a menace to the nurses.

On Friday 19th October, Dad began to hiccup. He stopped hiccupping on the morning of **Monday 22nd October 2001.** He stopped hiccupping, and died.

Paul had anticipated the worst and had flown over to arrive at Dads bedside just minutes before he gave up the ghost. And Hilary was there. Hilary had told me that things were looking terminal for Dad, so I'd hopped on my bike and raced up the road to be with Mum at home. I could hear the phone ringing as I approached Mum's door, and I tried to answer it before Mum could; but she beat me to it. It *was* Hilary. She told Mum that Dad was dead. This wasn't ideal, but had I not been there, it could've been much worse.

Mum was okay. I don't think it really sank in that Dad was gone forever. I don't think it ever did.

We now had a funeral to arrange, and it was going to be a big one. How would Mum cope?

Well-wishers began to appear at Mum's door later that afternoon. They needed entertained, the house needed tidied and the kitchen made ready for tea-making........ *And* we had to arrange Dad's funeral.

Good funeral directors are, in my experience, very thorough, very sympathetic, and very good at their job; just supply the dead person, and they'll do *everything*. And they *did* almost everything, and this allowed us to be with Mum.

Dad had been a well-known businessman in Bangor, chairman of numerous public committees, he had served high office on the borough council, he'd been a church elder, the district governor of the Rotary Club, and a Justice of the Peace: more people knew Dad than Dad knew people. His funeral was going to fill the church with hundreds of people, and we were naturally very worried about how Mum would cope.

As Hilary and my Claire helped to prepare Mum on the morning of the funeral they realised how much she had neglected her own personal hygiene. And they had a problem: Mum was infested with head lice – her head was Nit City, her hair was *alive* with them. They tried to clear Mum's head of the lice, but there were so many that nothing they tried had complete effectiveness. Our hearts sank at the realisation that we couldn't clear this infestation before the funeral, and we knew that Mum would greet everyone with a big hug, which would naturally give the lice ample opportunity to spread their circus far and wide (sorry about that, everyone).

The funeral went okay, as funerals go. Mum didn't become too distressed or too emotional, it was as if she wasn't a close relation to Dad, just a guest at the funeral of a friend of a friend. I don't know how many at the funeral knew about Mum's condition, it couldn't have been *that* many; they must have been impressed by how brave and cheerful Mum remained on such a difficult occasion.

Without Dad, Mum's condition seemed to plateau out a little. The stress of caring for Dad had gone, but she was still forgetful and making silly mistakes, however she wasn't affecting anyone else so this was okay–*ish*.

I fitted security lights to the front and rear of her house, and spy-holes to the doors. Another appointment with the mental health clinic could be arranged at short notice if I felt that Mum required another evaluation, but there was no additional concern to prompt this. (In fact I was rather hoping that now that Dad was gone, Mum might somehow be cured.)

Mum stayed with me that Christmas. Our new house was almost finished, and my Claire had insisted that we move in regardless. It was a mess of boxes, and stacked furniture, and books, and piles of children's stuff everywhere. And Mum clearly felt quite at home in this chaos.

I'd taken the plunge to begin to consolidate all of Mum and Dad's accounts and shares and savings into one place. Mum kept complaining about having no money, but the truth was that she had lots of money, but it was all over the place. It all needed sorted out anyway, but now that Dad was dead, I had the perfect excuse to *interfere* again to try to tidy this mess.

Twenty-nine, that's the number of financial institutions and accounts Dad had his money tied up with. It took months to identify, locate and sort them all, (and there's still a small one missing to this day). I sold their shares in this and that, closed accounts, cashed in savings plans, and eventually bunged the whole lot into two accounts at the bank: a current account, and a high-interest savings account, (I've explained this in one sentence – in reality it took me over two years of frustration, letter-writing, meetings, and more meetings with accountants and solicitors to consolidate all Mum's assets).

But I still hadn't managed to find the deeds to Mum's house.

I knew that if the deeds were in the house (which seemed the most likely place because no one else claimed to have them), I'd have to make the search in one big effort, because if I started and stopped, by the time I continued again Mum would most likely have moved more stuff around, so I'd have to start all over again. And the house was indescribably cluttered – *seriously*, you have no idea....

When Mum's mum died, she insisted on moving everything from granny's house into her own house; when Mum's aunt and uncle died, she did the same thing (it was easier that way, and it could all be sorted out *later*). Mum lived alone in a four-bedroom villa, *and there was no room in it*. The house had three houses of furniture in it, plus all the junk and stuff that people keep *just in case* (in case of what?). Every room was plied high with *stuff*. Everywhere, every horizontal space was piled high with more and more *stuff*, broken *stuff*, damaged *stuff*, *stuff* that the dog had begun to chew,..... Some of this *stuff* was important, needed to be found, sorted and filed. So the deeds remained missing.

On the bright side, Mum's brother had decided to retire from London to move closer to home. He was disabled and needed a little care, but his company and craic was great for Mum's spirits.

Dad's birthday came around. Mum remembered that. **16th April 2002**, she rose that morning and went from cluttered room to cluttered room looking for Dad to wish him happy birthday. She was very tearful by the time I called with her. Some of her friends called during the afternoon, and that helped distract her. Funny though, that she'd remember 16th April as Dad's birthday, but forget that he'd been buried six months earlier.

The quarterly visits to the psychiatrist continued, and we were buoyed by the previous professional suggestion that Mum's forgetful condition was improving since the stress of Dad's care had been lifted from her life. Mum was advised to aid her short-term memory by keeping a notebook in her pocket (Ha!), and keeping clutter to a minimum (Ah, ha ha ha ha ha ha.......).

STAGE 3 *with Hindsight*

Realising that Mum was forgetting things, *significant* things, was a worry for her family, of course it was. Telling Mum that she was forgetting things, and that she needed help, wasn't easy.

None of us like the thought of growing old, so denial is the first thing we do (illustrated in sales of Botox, and hair dye), but you can't disguise mental decline as easily as physical aging, you can only deny it.

It was incredibly embarrassing to have Mum's close friends phone me to ask what I was doing to help, (*if they only knew*). They were right to be worried for her, but they didn't understand the fine line that must be walked at this stage of dementia – you can't just take over; I had to be incredibly diplomatic and sensitive in the way in which arrangements were made and how changes (and my interference) were introduced.

Those friends of Mum's who understood her condition *were* very supportive to her – and this was important.

43

Without the support of her friends, without their frequent phone calls, and visits, and the socialising that they encouraged Mum to participate in, she would have been very isolated because she had begun to lose her motivation, (she might have become one of those crazy old people who collect cats).

If I analysed my whole involvement with Mum, this stage (Stage 3) is perhaps the stage where I made the most mistakes, ...where I have the most regrets. I tried, and I know I erred.

My biggest regret is that I hadn't realised how Mum's forgetfulness was negatively affecting Dad's quality of life. Nature would possibly have allowed Dad an earlier and dignified death in 1999, but Mum was naturally desperate to keep him alive, and she insisted on constant medical intervention to prolong his life unnaturally. Such a gentle gentleman did not deserve to suffer Mum's careless care, albeit with her best intentions.

But what should I have done ?

.......I'm incredibly sorry Dad.

STAGE FOUR

Moderate Cognitive Decline (Mild Dementia)

Clear-cut deficit on careful clinical interview.

Deficit manifest in following areas:

(a) decreased knowledge of current and recent events;

(b) may exhibit some deficit in memory of ones personal history;

(c) concentration deficit elicited on serial subtractions;

(d) decreased ability to travel, handle finances, etc.

Frequently no deficit in following areas:

(a) orientation to time and place;

(b) recognition of familiar persons and faces;

(c) ability to travel to familiar locations.

Inability to perform complex tasks. Denial is dominant defense mechanism. Flattening of affect and withdrawal from challenging situations frequently occur.

Global Deterioration Scale © Barry Reisberg, MD

Brian Bailie

STAGE 4 July 2002 – October 2002

Behaviour timeline:

* Mum's emotional rejection of her mental decline.
* Readily charmed by salesmen, (and agreeing to have renovations to the house).
* Steady increase in confusion.

Event timeline:

* Confirmation of Mum's regression with Alzheimer's.
* Taking full control of Mum's finances.
* (Against my better judgement) telling Mum that she had been diagnosed with Alzheimer's.
* Removal of Mum's driving licence.
* Realising that Mum needed proper fulltime supervision.

On 11th July 2002, one year to the day since her first visit to the mental health clinic, and I received confirmation of diagnosis: Mum is suffering with Alzheimer's disease.

I made arrangements with the bank that allowed me to write cheques from Mum's account (with Hilary's joint signature). Hilary found and took responsibility for Mum's pension book and the bankcards, and became more involved with the weekly grocery shopping.

And, against my better judgement, (but following the "expert" advice of Mum's psychiatrist), I told Mum that she had Alzheimer's disease.

When you think about it, this is just stupid, because it's going to be forgotten (isn't that the point of Alzheimer's?). This is one of those moments when I wish that I'd ignored expert advice; all I did was distress Mum to tears and fears. *What was the point?* I'd said this to the psychiatrist, but she insisted that this was an important element of Mum's acceptance of her condition. (I'd like to have given the quack a condition with the toe of my boot.)

A couple of weeks later I also had to bring up the subject of the car.

Mum loved driving. And I had to tell her that she couldn't drive anymore. This was almost as bad as telling her she had Alzheimer's. Her driving licence had expired. I reasoned with her that she didn't really need the car, so why reapply for another licence?

I knew that if she reapplied for a driving licence that there would be a standard medical question that would have to state her mental condition, (and the driver licensing agency would reply to inform her that she was forbidden to drive because of her Alzheimer's disease, thereby putting the diagnosis in print for her read over and over again).

When I told Mum that she couldn't drive, she became very upset. I had her car keys in my pocket, and her car was locked. She punched me in frustration, and she broke down in tears, again. (You're going to think this is mad, but the compromise I made was that Mum should keep her car. The car stayed parked in her drive, but she never drove it again. But it was *her* car, and it was parked in *her* drive, and Mum was happy. And I later insured Hilary to drive it, so Mum did still get the use of it, sort of.)

15th August 2002 Mum had another mental health appointment that revealed that her condition had advanced *significantly*, and the psychiatrist informed us that Mum wouldn't be safe living on her own for much longer. A nurse called with Mum each afternoon (if Mum was in) to make sure that she was taking all her medication, but apart from that, Mum was alone most of the day.

I tried an experiment: I tried working from Mum's house (I was getting naff-all done in my studio because I was spending most of my time with Mum – it was worth a try, I thought). So I took my notes and laptop, and established my-self in Mum's dining room with the hope of *being there* for her, and the vague intention of achieving some work. (If there's a job out there that involves having last week's news read aloud to you, and being fed copious amounts of biscuits and ice-cream, this plan would have been a roaring success), I got noth-ing done; I only amused Mum for a little while.

I'd asked for another psychiatrist to offer us a second opinion. It was to be an evaluation at Mum's house (in the hope that in familiar surroundings Mum would be more re-laxed and be able to answer the questions a little better). On 27th **August** I arrived for the meeting at Mum's house, Hilary arrived, the second psychiatrist arrived; but (despite phoning to remind her an hour earlier) Mum had forgotten, and gone out for coffee with her cousin. Another appointment was made for the 10th September.

I called with Mum on **30th August 2002**, having taken the long way home from a job in Armagh. My mouth dropped and my heart sank as I turned the corner. I was greeted by a gang of workmen who were just tidying up after having dug up the length of Mum's drive to install pipes from the road that connected the house to the natural gas supply, and they'd hammered the hell out of the kitchen to mount a great boiler on the wall. A layer of dust had settled on the piles of clutter and stuff that had been heaped about to let the workmen do their job. Mum was in fine fettle having been kept busy making hundreds of cups of tea for everyone all day, and the house was hot – like a flipp'n sauna. Oh, and among the dusty piles of stuff there was a bill for the installation - £1,800.

Stage 4, with Hindsight

I wish I'd never taken the psychiatrist's advice to tell Mum that she had Alzheimer's – I still regret that. It was stupid, distressing, and pointless.

It was fortunate that Mum's driving licence had expired, otherwise I wouldn't have had that valid opportunity to stop her from driving. Explaining the driving licence business was unpleasant but necessary in case she caused an accident (I have a good friend whose wife drove with Alzheimer's: she would forget to indicate, and forget where she'd parked, but most dangerously she forgot to use her windscreen wipers when it rained – so she couldn't see where she was going).

Mum could still be convincingly lucid, and most strangers never noticed anything peculiar about her behaviour. Whether salesmen took advantage of Mum at this stage cannot be proved, but it's obvious that she had become very gullible.

Sorting out Mum's money was a nightmare. Everything had to be done in writing because Mum couldn't understand enough long enough to speak to these institutions by phone.

This stage of Mum's decline was very frustrating for the family. We didn't know what to do, and the professional advice wasn't helpful. We had accepted that Mum was going to continue to decline to become less independent, more of a risk to herself, and more of a responsibility for us – and we *really* didn't know what we were doing.

.

STAGE FIVE

Moderately Severe Cognitive Decline (Moderate Dementia)

Patient can no longer survive without some assistance. Patient is unable during interview to recall a major relevant aspect of their current lives, e.g., an address or telephone number of many years, the names of close family members (such as grandchildren), the name of the high school or college from which they graduated.

Frequently some disorientation to time (date, day of week, season, etc.), or to place. An educated person may have difficulty counting back from 40 by 4s or from 20 by 2s.

Persons at this stage retain knowledge of many major facts regarding themselves and others. They invariably know their own names and generally know their spouse's and children's names. They require no assistance with toileting and eating, but may have some difficulty choosing the proper clothing to wear.

Global Deterioration Scale © Barry Reisberg, MD

STAGE 5 TIMELINE **October 2002 – January 2003**

Behaviour timeline:

* Inability to recognise danger or the need to take action.
* Complete forgetfulness of a recent visitor to the door.
* Increasingly childlike behaviour.

Event timeline:

* The decision to implement a plan to protect Mum from herself.
* The introduction of Mum's full-time daily care and companionship at home.

I returned from a week abroad on the **3ʳᵈ October 2002**, and called with Mum the next day. Hilary had called a few days earlier to take Mum to an ear appointment, and had arrived to discover Mum climbing out of the kitchen window, (she'd lost her key, again).

There was a leak in the bathroom. Water was dripping through the ceiling rose in the breakfast room. The ceiling was all bulged, pregnant with damp, and Mum was cheerfully collecting the dripping water in plastic buckets. She flicked the light switch on and off several times to prove to me that it was perfectly safe: there was a flash and a bang.

The cause was simple. The new water heating system had created too much pressure in the old lead pipe-work, and it had begun to leak under the strain. I isolated the light switch, and called a plumber who said he would call first thing the next day.

When I phoned next mid-morning, the plumber hadn't been, and the water was still drip, drip, dripping through the light fitting. I phoned the plumber and got no reply, so I phoned another plumber who said he'd be there within the hour. I arrived at Mum's at the same time as the plumber. He turned off the mains water supply to the house and said that he'd send a man round within the hour to replace the old leaking lead plumbing.

So far, so good, says I. And sure enough another plumber arrived, so I chivvied him up the stairs and set him straight to work in the bathroom.

And then *another* plumber arrived with all his tools and a vanload of pipes. Two plumbers? "Yes, my boss was just here and turned off your water. He's sent me round to replace all your old pipe-work". But,......? I asked the bloke upstairs who he was: "I'm the plumber you phoned yesterday. I called earlier but the dog wouldn't let me in, so I told your mother I'd come back later". Mum had completely forgotten a visit from the first plumber when her dog went berserk only an hour or so earlier – forgotten, like it never happened.

Money is a wonderful thing for sorting out misunderstandings. I paid one plumber to go away, and the other plumber to stay and complete the work. I'm not sure which was which, but they were both happy (if a little confused), and the drip stopped.

It was decision time *again*. It was obvious now that Mum couldn't be left alone in the house during the day. She was losing keys, money, cheque books, she was eating dog biscuits, climbing out of windows, and she'd had managed to set fire to the porch (which only resulted in scorch damage, but it could've been much, much worse).

I'd asked my accountant to look at Mum's situation, and he wasn't impressed. He reckoned that a care home would be at least £12,000 a year, and Mum could easily live another ten to fifteen years. But we needed to make a plan and take action in the near future.

57

Hilary mentioned that there was a possibility that she could take a career-break from her job. When she confirmed that this option was available to her, we didn't take too long to think about it; Hilary agreed to be Mum's daytime carer companion for the twelve months of her maximum permitted break. I arranged that Hilary would be paid the same amount as she was presently earning so that she wouldn't suffer any financial loss, (and this compensation could be made as a gift, and tax-free after seven years, my accountant explained).

Hilary began work as Mum's full-time caring companion on **22nd October 2002**, (one full year to the day since Dad had died).

Hilary's companionship duties made Mum much more dependent. Hilary became the mother, Mum was the naughty child. I know it was difficult for Hilary, because she told me so. She had to do everything for Mum: bathe her, dress her, feed her, and accompany her everywhere during the day. (But it also allowed me to get on a little more effectively with what was left of my little business.)

The bank found the deeds to Mum's house. It was a full year since I'd originally asked them, since they'd assured me that they didn't have them. And they'd had them all the time. They apologised. I seethed with relief.

Amazingly I hadn't managed to complete the Power of Attorney for Mum. The solicitors had been *really* dragging their heels for months about this, finding little problems here, and delays there. I don't know why this was so difficult for them; it was as if they didn't trust me with Mum's care and best interests. I phoned the psychiatrist to confirm if Mum was still legally suitable to sign her name on these documents in a brief moment of lucidity, with witnesses. When I received the okay on this, the solicitors delayed again saying, "Really? Can we have that in writing?" *What was the problem?*

The solicitors then seemed to run out of delaying tactics until I received a letter from them stating that they'd had a burglary and arson attack (I know it's extreme, but I did wonder at the authenticity of this event), and *then* they suggested that I might want to take Mum's legal work elsewhere.

So I asked Mum to sign a letter to her solicitors instructing them to hand over all of her business to *my* solicitor.

But when I presented this letter to them, they refused to hand over Mum's files stating that they couldn't release the files until her account had been settled in full, but her account couldn't be billed until they'd have time to calculate their expenses to date.

I arrived at the solicitors' offices and politely asked for all of Mum's files. I told them that I'd settle their account in full by return of post as soon as they managed to make time to send it to me; and I explained that they knew where Mum lived, and that she wasn't going to run away without paying them (this, to a firm who had been our family solicitors for perhaps fifty years). I removed the boxes of files and deposited them with *my* solicitor, and started over again. (And though it galled me to do it, I did pay the dismissed solicitors by return of post, even though my solicitor argued that Mum was being overcharged for work that had clearly not been completed.)

I also appointed *my* accountant to be Mum's accountant, and with the full approval of Paul and Hilary, I instructed the accountant to create an estate plan that would protect Mum's assets in the best possible way. And, although Dad had been dead for over a year, we agreed to the accountant's recommendation of a Deed of Variation to Dad's will, which would protect Mum from a very nasty tax bill.

STAGE 5 *with Hindsight*

This stage of Mum's mental decline could have been much more distressing if Hilary hadn't been able to take that twelve-month career break. Without Hilary's career break, Mum would have been institutionalised prematurely, at a stage in her decline when she needed supervision and assistance, but she didn't need locked up. But without Hilary, Mum *would have been* locked up, because what other practical options were available to us?

I hate to bring this up (because Mum would scold me for suggesting that we were anything other than *her* children), but I did wonder if the solicitor was dragging his heels over Mum's affairs because he knew that we were adopted children. Did he doubt that I had anything but the very best intentions for Mum? Mum and Dad are the only mum and dad we three have ever known (and we're the only children Mum and Dad ever had), and it's reasonably insulting to think that other

61

people might have imagined our motives to be mercenary. Anyway, the legal work was late, and becoming later, and I couldn't risk Mum's future financial security by allowing it to become *too* late. Without the completion of this work Mum would have been left vulnerable in so many ways. It is an essential part of the long-term care of a loved one. It's unpleasant and tedious work, but it's essential that it be completed correctly and efficiently (by professionals who realise the importance and urgency of such matters).

STAGE SIX.

Severe Cognitive Decline (Moderately Severe Dementia)

May occasionally forget the name of the spouse upon whom they are entirely dependent for survival. Will be largely unaware of all recent events and experiences in their lives. Retain some knowledge of their past lives but this is very sketchy. Generally unaware of their surroundings, the year, the season, etc.

May have difficulty counting from 10, both backward and, sometimes, forward. Will require some assistance with activities of daily living, e.g., may become incontinent, will require travel assistance but occasionally will be able to travel to familiar locations. Diurnal rhythm frequently disturbed. Almost always recall their own name. Frequently continue to be able to distinguish familiar from unfamiliar persons in their environment.

Personality and emotional changes occur. These are quite variable and include:

(a) delusional behavior, e.g., patients may accuse their spouse of being an impostor, may talk to imaginary figures in the environment, or to their own reflection in the mirror;

(b) obsessive symptoms, e.g., person may continually repeat simple cleaning activities;

(c) *anxiety symptoms, agitation, and even previously nonexistent violent behavior may occur;*

(d) *cognitive abulla, i.e., loss of willpower because an individual cannot carry a thought long enough to determine a purposeful course of action.*

Global Deterioration Scale © Barry Reisberg, MD

STAGE 6 TIMELINE   **January 2003 – March 2010**

Behaviour timeline:

* Mum's growing dependency on her carer.
* Full acceptance of role reversal of parent and child.
* Period of unprovoked sporadic aggression.
* Habitual incontinence.
* Childish behaviour.
* Need for constant supervision for the most basic of tasks.
* Mum would 'switch off' when she was alone and unstimulated.
* Dental care issues.
* Loss of appetite.
* Total inability to perform a familiar, simple task without supervision.
* Mum becomes unstable on her feet and a danger to herself.
* Mum's susceptibility to motion-sickness.
* Falling out of bed.
* Grinding her teeth.

Event timeline:

* Planning the transition to permanent care-home accommodation.
* Completion of Mum's financial and legal affairs.
* Introducing Mum to day-care.
* Seeking suitable residential care.
* Removing Mum to a residential care-home.

- Selling Mum's house.
- The realisation that Mum had become a business to me.
- Doctor prescribes sedatives to prevent Mum from falling.
- Seeking a suitable nursing home.
- Identifying unnecessary drugs, and beginning to wean Mum from them.
- Noticing Mum's neglect under new nursing home management.
- Moving Mum to a new nursing home.
- Removal of Mum's all of teeth.

By **January 2003**, Mum's estate planning seemed to be nearing completion by the joint efforts of her newly appointed solicitor and accountant. And Hilary was finding that being Mum's full-time caring companion was physically and emotionally draining. Mum was becoming more and more difficult, less and less predictable, and more and more dependent.

It was at this stage that Mum became sporadically aggressive. She would suddenly punch Hilary from behind, or grit her teeth as she twisted a nasty pinch on Hilary's arm. All without any kind of provocation – she'd just do it, and then forget that she'd done it.

And Mum had become consistently incontinent. Her bed needed changed every morning. I'd removed the dishwasher from Mum's kitchen and replaced it with a tumble-dryer to help with the increasing daily washing routine; it wasn't much, but it was all I could think of to help at the time.

By the beginning of **February 2003** Mum lost her sporadic aggression, and she became very child-like.

She would run over to a pram in the street and stick her head in to *koochey-koochey-koo* at the baby; she would run after dogs (especially puppies) in the same manner and try to pick them up for a cuddle. Hilary had to double-check where Mum was when she called her for a bath, because Mum would just strip off all her clothes wherever she happened to be (the kitchen, the garden, anywhere).

Unsupervised, Mum would dress like a toddler, all inside out and back-to-front; she would eat lunch, and then start making lunch again. And she would disclose inappropriate secrets: Mum casually explained to Hilary how *that* couple aren't happy because *he* can't make an erection; and one afternoon she had been chatting with an elderly gentleman on the high street, and when she'd said her goodbyes, Mum turned to Hilary all matter of fact and said, "That was Paul's uncle." Hilary was understandably dumbfounded and embarrassed by some of the things Mum was disclosing. If Mum thought something, she'd just come straight out and say it, like the time they were walking along the beach, and when a passer-by commented on how chilly the weather was, Mum replied, "Yes isn't it – I thought I'd no knickers on." (I'm sure that brightened someone's day.)

Mum's condition was becoming more obvious to her friends. If someone had brought Mum back from being out, as Mum removed her coat in the hall she'd forget whether she was removing her coat, or putting it on, and she'd ask, "Where are we going, again?" Twice, Mum had been invited to a friend's house for lunch, Hilary had collected her to bring her home after the lunch, and Mum then phoned her friend to explaine that she couldn't come for lunch today because she was feeling a little tired – just like that, almost immediate complete forgetfulness of a significant event.

Mum greeted Hilary each morning like they were long lost friends. Mum would ask Hilary why she wasn't at work today, and Hilary always explained that she'd just taken that day off, to which Mum exclaimed, "Och, that's lovely dear, come on in" (_every_ day). Hilary prepared Mum's lunch each day, and then left her alone to eat it; when Hilary returned half an hour later, again Mum would greet Hilary like she hadn't seen her for months, and Hilary would have to explain again that she'd just taken a day off work to visit her, ...

As Mum became less aggressive and more childlike, Hilary became more settled with her responsibilities.

At Mum's next visit to the psychiatrist on 27th **February 2003**, Hilary asked about Mum's care after October (when Hilary would have to return to her career). We agreed a plan to introduce Mum to day-care at a specialised care unit, and gradually build up these visits from once, to several visits each week, so that by October Mum would be accustomed to that type of environment, and (if it was appropriate) a future move to permanent care would be less traumatic. That was the idea, and it seemed to be a sensible one.

Finally, by the 9th **March 2003** Mum's estate planning, and Dad's Deed of Variation, and a new will for Mum had been completed to the satisfaction of the extended family and professional advisors.

I know: you're thinking that there's no way Mum would know what the blazes she was signing – it couldn't possibly be legal, could it? Well I double-checked with Mum's psychiatrist, and we were told that because Mum had known about the intentions of the planned arrangements, and because everything was in Mum's best interests, provided that it was clarified again to her in a moment of lucidity in front of independent witnesses of professional standing, Mum *could* sign the documents and it *would* be legal. The only person who could object to Mum signing these documents would be HM Inspector of Taxes; however everything was done correctly, and now that it had been completed I had assured Mum's financial security and her future ability to afford the level of care she deserved for the rest of her life.

The **24th June 2003** was a big day for Hilary. It should have been a big day for Mum, but we don't think she noticed. This was Mum's first afternoon at the day-care centre, and at almost 71 Mum was the youngest patient there. Hilary and I had visited the facilities a week earlier to inspect it and get a feel for the staff and the general mood of the other patients. It wasn't what we wanted for Mum, *day-care* that is, but as daycare facilities go, this was nice and we knew that Mum *should* enjoy it.

Hilary was naturally very apprehensive about Mum first visit to an institution. She phoned to check on Mum mid-afternoon, and heard her laughing and joking in the background. Mum knit, she sang songs, she played games and had a great time; and when it came time to leave, Mum hugged everyone on her way out. Success. Success because Mum was convinced that she was only there to help look after the confused old people – but it didn't matter, Mum had gone without a fuss, made friends and thoroughly enjoyed herself.

I phoned Mum later that evening to ask how the day had gone for her. But she replied saying that she didn't know what she would be doing today, and that she was waiting to have breakfast with Hilary.

This unawareness of time became more of an issue in the summer months when dawn is early and dusk is late. In good weather a June day can be eighteen hours of bright blue-skies, and often Hilary would arrive in the morning to find Mum sitting motionless on a kitchen stool, head bowed and hands together, just staring at the floor like a robot on flat batteries.

By **August 2003** Hilary and I knew that we were going to have to become more proactive about securing full-time residential care for Mum in the near future.

Mum was still going once a week to the day-centre at the local care unit (to help, as Mum believed), and we made enquiries about securing a place for Mum on the waiting list for their residential section, which specialised in the care of patients with Alzheimer's disease.

Late August I replaced Mum's bed. I took the old one out and dumped it, and replaced it with one of the many others in her house. By this stage Mum wasn't even undressing for bed. I had arranged for a nurse to call with her in the evening to help prepare her for bed, but now Mum was barricading herself in the house once Hilary had left, and the nurses simply couldn't get in – key, or no key. So this meant that Mum was unsupervised (and effectively inaccessible). And she was going to bed with all her clothes on, with the dog on top for added protection; and she'd pee herself before morning. This meant hours of washing routine, *every* day.

Hilary and I had taken obvious precautions to avoid potential disasters: removed the plug fuse from the toaster, the clothes iron, and the kettle; and we'd disconnected the gas stove so she could only heat food with the microwave or electric oven. We had also removed all the coal from the house (not that it was ever cold since it had been plumbed directly into a rig in the North Sea for it's gas heating), but with an open hearth in the house, and the habit of always lighting a fire for company when the weather was poor, there remained a real risk that Mum would attempt to light *something*.

Hilary replaced the fuse in the iron each day to do the laundry. Mum *loved* ironing at this stage. She used to *hate* ironing, but now she would spend hours and hours ironing the same folded sheet, over and over, and over, loving every smooth moment of it.

By **mid-September 2003** I'd agreed a care package for Mum that included four nursing calls every day (if Mum let them in). And all her meals were delivered, ready to reheat.

She had become less and less predictable, and she'd stopped caring practically for her dog – simple things, like letting the animal out to toilet itself. If Mum had overfed the dog (which was normal), and if its pleas for outdoor relief had been ignored, by the time a visitor called, the dog would be so desperate it would shoot out the open door like a ballistic missile primed to explode on contact with grass, (the dog was spoilt, untrained, ruled Mum's house, was fat like a fluffy balloon with legs, noisy and smelly, and generally very unlikeable – but we did feel sorry for the old thing).

By **9th October 2003** Mum was assessed to be officially "At Risk" to herself. Her need for Housing with Care was deemed "Critical" by her doctor, psychiatrist, and nurses, (and her family couldn't disagree).

We phoned the residential care section of the day-care centre where Mum had been visiting each week, and explained Mum's situation. Coincidentally, a room would be available for Mum the next morning. And just like that, everything was finalised. Hilary and I felt pleased and relieved, but mostly we felt shock.

I think Hilary found Mum's incarceration the most difficult because she'd been used to spending all day, every day with Mum.

As usual, Hilary took Mum to the day-care section of the home. Then Hilary returned to help me gather up clothes and bedding, and a bed, and bits of furniture, and paintings and a rug, and bits and pieces to prepare her new room, (her new home).

Once we'd furnished Mum's room, and tidied away all her clothes and toiletries, we left. At the end of the day-care session Mum was casually escorted into the main building and shown her room. Familiar objects and photographs surrounded her, and she had no bother accepting her new accommodation.

We'd thought that Mum would've made a scene, gone looking for her fat dog, wrestled with the carers, cried to be let out, but no – it couldn't have gone smoother. Mum accepted things as if she'd always lived there. The only people left traumatised by the resettlement seemed to be Hilary and me.

It's a big, big thing to put your parent into a care home. It's a big, big thing.

I was away on business the week after Mum entered the home. This gave me time to reflect a little and appreciate things from a distance. Now that Mum had left home there was a mammoth task that had to be undertaken sooner or later, a task that I'd managed to put off until now: Clearing Mum's house. It was a monumental undertaking: three house-fuls of *everything* in one house, and it would have to be done thoroughly and correctly, pile by pile, drawer by drawer, shelf by shelf, room by room. My heart sank. I'd think about it later....

In **December 2003** Mum was still enjoying her new home and new routine. She was blissfully very happy and un-inhibited, and she'd do the silliest childish things. She would prance about and dance about, she'd wear her knickers on her head to have a straight-faced conversation, and she'd dress her-self with skirts over slacks, and *always* carry her handbag.

That handbag needed a health warning. It contained the most surprising and horrible things: bras, pants (fresh and not so fresh), tissues (used and unused), false teeth (hers, and others'), spectacles (again, hers and others'), bits of toast (with and without marmalade), pieces of cake and biscuits, and any-thing else she might find lying about the place. It smelt like a dog's dinner.

Hilary and I visited Mum anytime we were passing, but Wednesday morning became our regular morning with Mum, and we'd take her to the shopping mall with her brother to browse the shops and visit a café for elevenses. (And although things have changed a lot for all of us, ever since then Wednesday morning remains our morning rendezvous with Mum.)

In late **December 2003** I made an appointment for an estate agent to call to offer me some advice about preparing Mum's house for sale. I knew that the kitchen was a disaster and needed ripped out and replaced, the bathroom wasn't much better, most of the windows needed replacing, and the whole place was long overdue a coat of paint (all these things would've been near-impossible while Mum was living there). I still struggled with the thought of the clearance and sale of Mum's house. It didn't feel right. But of course it was the only sensible thing to be done with the place.

Paul visited that Christmas. My Claire was six-months pregnant, but we'd arranged for Christmas dinner at our house, and Mum and her brother, and Paul and his wife were all invited. Despite the fact that Paul would be driving past Mum's home, (and it would be a ninety-minute round-trip for me, twice), I volunteered to collect Mum and take her home again because I knew that Paul would've been trauma-tised by her condition since he last saw her, and he just wouldn't have been prepared for her unpredictable and unin-hibited behaviour. The day went well and without incident. It was sad that family circumstances had suffered such a sea-change from the Christmases we all remembered.

After Christmas I accepted that it was silly to keep postponing the sale of Mum's house: she'd never be returning to it. So having spent an hour one day and couple of hours the next, and making almost no progress, I decided to commit to clearing Mum's house properly, and just consider it a fulltime job until it was completed. Day after day after dirty, dusty, backbreaking day I spent going through everything, item by item.

I hate clearing other people's stuff. I've done it for four dead relations, and it's one of the most horrible things. You've got to sort through personal things, private and inti-mate things, letters and photographs and collections, and things that you know had close sentimental value for them. But what value does it have now? Does anyone in the family want it? Does it have any resale value? Would a charity shop be interested? If *you* kept it, where would you put it? One man's treasure is another man's junk, but which is which? We come into this world with nothing, and we leave it the same way, why do we surround ourselves with so much *stuff*?

But y'know, the worst clearance I've ever done will always be clearing Mum's stuff: because she wasn't dead, she was about three minutes away, innocently frolicking about the care home, and there was I going through all her stuff (and all the stuff Mum had taken from Granny's house clearance, and all the stuff she had taken from her uncle and aunt's house clearance, yes: *three* housefuls of stuff), and I genuinely felt like a burglar, like I was intruding, worse than naughty. You'll not understand unless you've had to do it – it's *truly* horrible.

Slowly I began to see progress in my sorting and clearing, (although I was miserable with my acute allergy to house dust). I'd sorted piles and piles for the dump, piles and piles for the charity shops, several piles for the second-hand bookshop, and a pile for the antique dealers. Big things, like the piano and tables and beds and paintings were distributed among the extended family and Mum's close friends. But it still felt like I was stealing.

I hired a van, and Hilary and I removed the sorted piles of everything from the house. Afterwards, we looked around the empty rooms and I guess we were both thinking the same thing: What if Mum gets cured? What if she gets better and decides to come home? It's all gone! And this thought takes a long time to go away. This thought was constantly on my mind as I arranged the sale of Mum's house. She loved that house; she loved the unbroken views across Belfast Lough to the green hills of Antrim, the changing moods of the sea, and the familiar distant shadow of the Mull of Kintyre. And now I was stealing that from her too. So, much as I wanted a cure for Mum, I was now really worried in case she *did* recover.

I washed and vacuumed the whole house and had it all smelling of cleaning products before the Sale signs went up front and back on **17th January 2004**. Apart from everything else, I reckon I'd removed about one-and-a-half tonnes of rubbish to the dump – at least that.

I was hoping that the house wouldn't sit too long unsold. As it turned out we had a bidding war between determined buyers from all over the UK. There were so many enquiries that the estate agent decided to arrange an open day at the house for people to view it. It sold within the month for well above the original asking price.

Throughout 2004, while I was *still* busy tying up loose ends with solicitors and accountants, Mum was settled – *very* settled.

Hilary and I and Mum's brother continued our weekly Wednesday morning excursions with Mum. Some of Mum's friends would occasionally call with her, or take her out places for lunch or coffee. One of Mum's closest friends told me that she'd taken her to the cinema one afternoon, and when she took her back to the care home, Mum gave her friend a big hug and told her that she was happy there, had made lots of new friends, and that she shouldn't worry about her. So, it seemed that Mum understood something of what was happening, more than any of us were aware.

Mum's brother always tagged along with anyone he knew was visiting Mum. He could easily get a taxi to visit

Mum, or walk there on a good day. But I don't think I understood why he needed company until much later. Mum's brother had known and loved her all his life, and watching her like this was breaking his heart. He *couldn't* visit on his own; he needed the moral support of others to cope with seeing his big sister suffering this dementia. Mum's cousins also had great difficulty visiting her too. In fact, several of them have never visited her, and I fully understand: their hearts were broken, because *their* mother had suffered dementia, and so they knew all about it, and they simply couldn't bear to see Mum going the same way.

Mum was living in the present, she was living in a state of *now*. Things that happened last week, or yesterday, or a few minutes ago, had been completely deleted from her memory. But her memory was being deleted in reverse, like a candle slowly burning down to the base. Mum could talk at length and with great clarity about people and events from her distant past, of when she was a wee girl, like it was yesterday.

To be honest, (because of all the estate planning and constant meetings with solicitors and accountants, and social workers and doctors, and then the house clearance, and the house sale, and more and more meetings and decisions to be agreed and implemented, and so on and so forth) Mum had become a business to me. My career had all but stopped; I was struggling to play catch-up in the early mornings and late into the night, because Mum's affairs took up most of almost every weekday.

(I often wonder what the difference would've been for my wee business if I hadn't been distracted with Mum and Dad, and it's impossible to say – does it really matter?)

I didn't enjoy Mum and Dad being a business to me. In fact, it wasn't until the third anniversary of Dad's death that I realised that I'd not grieved for him – there had been so much to do and get done, his death was just another project to complete on top of looking after Mum. And that's not right; it really shouldn't be that way.

Accepting that Mum's regression was a one-way journey, I wanted to have some sort of a gathering for her. It has always annoyed me that the only time family and friends gather together is at weddings and funerals – especially funerals (where you don't need an invitation). And I realised that there was a real risk of this happening with Mum.

June 6ᵗʰ 2004 was the 50ᵗʰ anniversary of the Normandy D-Day Landings, and there were lots of things going on to commemorate that event locally and internationally, in the all the press and television news. And I decided that I'd use this highly publicised anniversary to organise a family and friend party for Mum – a date they'd definitely remember.

I booked a large function room and catering for at least a hundred people at the Old Inn at Crawfordsburn. It wasn't cheap, I didn't expect it to be, but as the last party Mum would probably ever have, I really didn't care about cost.

Hilary and I invited all of Mum's friends and family to join us, and asked that they share our invitation with any other friends of Mum's that we may have unintentionally omitted; and I specified no gifts, no flowers, no cards – it was just a big "At Home" and *everyone* was welcome.

I'm so pleased that we had that party for Mum. Her cousins were there whom she hardly ever saw; friends from her childhood school, Friend's School, Lisburn; friends from church; family and friends flew in from England and Scotland,

and Paul arrived from Bermuda. Everyone who was invited, came; no one made excuses.

Mum hugged and welcomed and hugged again every-one – she was in her element. Whether she genuinely recog-nised every face is irrelevant; the shared emotion was love. That party was such an overwhelming display of love and af-fection towards Mum – why don't we do this more often? (oh yeah, the cost). We really shouldn't wait until the person we love is dead before we gather to demonstrate our affection – that's just way too late.

By **September 2004** Mum's teeth *really* needed atten-tion. She had the breath of death, like vomit. But ever since Mum had been a wee girl she'd had this fear of dentists (so much so that I'd been told about her as a teenager kicking the dentist off his chair as he was working on her).

A good friend of mine is a dentist in Scotland; I asked him if he could recommend a local dentist who would be understanding with Mum's condition. I bit the bullet and made an appointment with this recommended friend of a friend. I recognised him from school, (in fact his father was the teacher who had kicked me out of Art class, and I'd unwillingly ended up studying Greek for two years). He was very good with Mum; he was *very* good. Mum was very nervous, very agitated, and very apprehensive; but the dentist played along with Mum's extreme condition of confused panic and nonsensical conversation to patiently complete a very gentle and diplomatically executed examination. Mum needed some work done, and a new plate made.

This dental work took weeks to complete because of Mum's condition. I made a standing appointment each Tuesday morning with the dentist, and gradually he completed the work over the course of the next five weeks.

Apart from the dental work, there's not much else to say about Mum's condition for the next few months. I'm sure she was getting worse, but Hilary and I were seeing her too frequently to notice small changes. Others noticed, others who hadn't seen Mum for several months; they were sometimes shocked by Mum's appearance or her total inability to recall who these well-meaning visitors might be.

If the weather was bad, or Hilary and I couldn't take Mum out on Wednesday morning, we'd just stay at the care-home and entertain her with chat, and dander about hand-in-hand visiting the other residents in the different wings (and she would introduce me to her friends as her *brother*). An easy way to focus Mum was an old picture book of Bangor. I could show Mum a picture on one page for her to point out this and that before I'd turn to the next page for her to do the same again; and then I'd return to the previous page, and she'd look at it afresh and begin the same conversation over again, like she'd never seen it before. And this could've gone on all day.

Mum became noticeably thin, so on **16th August 2005** the doctor prescribed Prednisolone. In fact Mum had become so thin that her engagement ring had slipped off her finger. I'd no idea what this drug was, I just trusted the doctor's judgement; apparently it's a steroid developed for the treatment of inflammation, arthritis, and allergies; weight gain is only a side effect. I asked Mum if she would let me look after her eternity ring, and she casually slipped it off her finger to give it to me. (The engagement ring was eventually discovered by a cleaner under Mum's bed.)

Curiously, Hilary and I were visiting Mum on the 3rd November when she wiggled her wedding ring off her finger, reached over to Hilary and quite deliberately gave it to her. I was pleased at this because it saved everyone from another game of Hunt the Ring. But Hilary's face went white when she read the inscription engraved on the inside of Mum's ring, it had the wedding date, 3rd November, 1955. That ring had been on Mum's finger for exactly fifty years, and she just popped it off and handed it to Hilary like she was supposed to, yet there is *no way* Mum could've known the date that day (and *that's* spooky).

I took Mum for a routine dental appointment at the end of **October 2005**. We suspected an abscess. Mum's kind and gentle dentist took a look at it and decided that it would be better for her to be treated at the hospital, discreetly explaining that, "She might need to be restrained."

Hospital,........ oh, goody.

The hospital dental appointment was for **21st November 2005**. I reckoned on this being a long day, so I took the precaution of asking one of the female employees from the care-home to accompany me in case Mum needed toileting. (As it turned out Mum didn't need the toilet, but it wasn't something I was prepared to risk on my own; I mean, which toilet do I take her into?)

The good news is that Mum was great at waiting – she just nodded off to sleep within minutes of sitting down in the waiting room. We were eventually called, examined quickly and sent for an X-ray. I was already sighing to myself – this was going to be *fun*.

Sure enough Mum was asked to stand still while a machine revolved around her head to make the X-ray image, and sure enough Mum refused to remain still while all this happened, three times. The technician eventually agreed to let me stand in with Mum to try to keep her still, so I was dressed in a great lead apron to give it a fourth attempt. The technician must have been pleased to see the back of us, because he sent us back to the dental department with a blurred X-ray of Mum's head (sounds about right). But the dentist demanded a proper X-ray, and sent us back round to try an X-ray with a standard plate image.

Mum sat down in a chair beside this great beast of an X-ray machine, and the technician swung round the back-plate vertically against the left side of Mum's head, and then targeted the X-ray generator at her right-hand side. Again, after a couple of failed attempts, the technician agreed to let me stay with Mum; I was dressed in lead again, and asked to gently hold Mum's head against the back-plate. Success: *finally* a result.

The successful X-ray offered a clear image of Mum's head with my hand where her brain should be. I loved the metaphor. It looked like her memory was waving goodbye. I asked if I could have a copy, (unfortunately the NHS isn't *that* obliging.)

Mum's brother died unexpectedly **12th April 2006**. Mum never noticed that he wasn't with us any Wednesday after that – never noticed, never asked about him. Hilary and I noticed; our mood was very low.

Mum's condition had seemed to level off over these years in the care-home. No significant deterioration, or if there *was* a big shift in her mood or memory, it would swing back again within a day or two.

One very simple task that Mum had forgotten was how to get into a car. She would stand on the doorframe and look over the top of the car as if she was supposed to climb onto the roof-rack, or she would try entering the car headfirst like she was climbing into a small cave. It was all very strange, and seatbelts were a complete confusion for her.

In **July 2007** Mum tripped and fell at the shopping mall with my Claire.

Then on **29th August 2007** I was informed that Mum had fallen out of bed during the night. She wasn't complaining about being sore or anything, but she looked like she'd been hit by a truck. Her face was badly bruised like an old banana, and she'd chipped one of her front teeth. Yet she remained cheerfully unaware that she'd been injured.

I didn't believe that she had fallen out of bed because she was sleeping in one of my big kids beds that had high sides at the head end that prevents falling out. I think Mum had got up in the night, stumbled, and banged her face on the dresser.

The fact was that Mum was becoming unsteady on her feet. We wanted to continue our Wednesday outings with her because we felt that these were important, but we had to cling onto her, one on each arm, or put her in a wheelchair, (but she never liked the wheelchair, it made her nervous).

By **mid-November 2007** Mum had become much more inactive and unresponsive. Only a couple of weeks earlier I'd been with her as she acted the lig and danced about the place. But now she just sat silently in an overly relaxed posture, oblivious to the world. She *would* eventually respond

91

with a big smile after a lot of coaxing, but she was noticeably beginning to withdraw into herself.

12th December 2007 Mum fell again. She'd had a visit from an old family friend, and he told me that Mum began to act silly and prance about the place like a wee girl. She fell over face-first and split her nose.

By **January 2008** Mum was spending most of her time sitting alone in her room ignoring the television that blared and glared by her side. I was told that she had become uneasy on her feet, and it now took two carers to help Mum walk; however because the care home was a little short-staffed after the New Year holidays, Mum had been allowed to vegetate alone in her room. With hindsight I can see that this wasn't quite true: why couldn't they just tell me that they had sedated Mum for her own protection? I'd have accepted *that*. I don't find lying acceptable (what else have they lied to me about?). They had controlled Mum's prancing about (which is acceptable to a point, I suppose, because they may have had Health and Safety issues had Mum fallen and injured herself or another resident), but as a side effect of this control measure they had turned Mum into a vegetable.

The doctor (who must have prescribed the sedative) explained that Mum "was degenerating naturally." I should've smacked him, the lazy lying locum.

Hilary and I began to look for alternative care for Mum. But waiting lists for nursing homes were long, *very* long. It could take maybe a year or more to be offered a place in a nursing home, and we knew that we'd probably have to accept the first place offered to us, regardless of how we liked or disliked it.

My Claire's sister, Janet, had recently returned to Northern Ireland to manage a private nursing home in Bangor, and I spoke to her for some advice. Janet had known Mum from before her dementia had started, and although the waiting list for the private nursing home she managed was thirty names long, she offered to give Mum first refusal on the next available place. It couldn't have been better, (of course I felt guilty about queue-jumping), but it *couldn't* have been better. Hilary and I visited Janet's nursing home. It was an unimpressive building, however the residents were in good spirits, and Janet had the place shipshape, with good morale among the staff.

As we waited for a place to become available for Mum at Janet's nursing home, I began to realise that helpless old people are really just a commodity. They are lumps of meat, cared for for cash. And I was part of this process, because in that nursing-home was a human being who would have to die before Mum could move in. And sooner or later someone who also wanted a place in that nursing home would be waiting for my Mum to die.

By **23ʳᵈ January 2008** a place had become available, and we moved Mum to Janet's nursing home.

Mum had a surprise for us. She hadn't been in the car for a couple of months because of her weakened condition, and unknown to us, she'd also become very susceptible to motion sickness. Within a minute of driving, Mum's mouth opened and her stomach contents were sprayed across the dashboard and controls of my car. Hilary reached round from behind with a handy plastic bag, but it was too late. Putrid lumpy yellow sticky acrid vomit was all over Mum and all over my left-arm and leg; Hilary and I were heaving with the stench, trying not to join in. I had to continue to drive (using a gearstick that now resembled a melting toffee apple). It was horrific. We were traumatised. Mum was smiling.

When we arrived, I peeled myself from the stinking car, and all I could do was laugh about it with Hilary. That was the longest two miles of my life.

We got cleaned up, washed Mum, and got her settled in to her new home.

Over the next few days Janet kept me up to date with everything. Mum was receiving much more attention in the nursing home, and she was responding very positively. The car-sickness had exhausted her a little, but apart from that, Mum's mood had improved significantly and she was smiling much more often, probably in response to the increase in personal attention from the staff.

Janet brought to my attention Mum's medications. She said that Mum had been prescribed an anti-psychotic drug that, in *her* professional opinion, wasn't appropriate for a person in Mum's condition. She asked me my permission to wean Mum off this drug with the doctor's consent, explaining that it could take about a year to complete this weaning process. Of course I wanted Mum off any drugs that were negatively affecting her quality of life, and I gave Janet the go-ahead to contact the doctor and begin the process immediately.

Mum appeared to be much happier under Janet's management in the nursing home. Her mood would continue to swing from bright and responsive to blank and unresponsive. But her good days were very good. We were all much happier.

On **11th July 2008** one of Mum's carers noticed her wincing as she was being dressed. Suspecting a break, Janet had one of her staff accompany Mum to hospital in an ambulance, (and they sat in A&E for ten hours awaiting treatment, surrounded by the usual victims of Northern Irish 12th July overindulgence), (and knowing Mum's tendency for redecorating the inside of moving vehicles, this must have been as traumatic for the young carer as it was exhausting for Mum). By the time Hilary and I saw Mum again, her arm had been plastered from fingers to bicep. Yet despite her discomfort it was obvious that Mum didn't notice (or remember) her broken arm, she just smiled as usual. But Hilary and I weren't smiling; we knew that a broken bone requires check-up appointments at the hospital, replacement casts and whatnot – and all of this meant putting our projectile-vomiting mum into a vehicle to make these routine return trips to the hospital.

How Mum broke her arm remains a mystery. It was a typical 'fall on outstretched hand' break. But Mum had a pressure mat beside her bed to alert staff if she attempted to get out of bed, and this hadn't activated, and none of the night staff said that they had noticed Mum out of bed; so we had to assume that Mum's bones had become weak and brittle, and that the break had been caused by moving about her bed in her sleep (maybe whacking the wall in her sleep?). Since Mum had moved to the nursing home her weight had increased by 14 pounds, so perhaps this *was* a possibility.

Hilary and I decided to take turns driving Mum to her hospital appointments. Since my car had been sprayed with vomit the last time, it was Hilary's turn to drive. We were well prepared with plastic bags, and dozens of towels and baby-wipes. And Janet had given Mum anti-sickness tablets a few hours before we departed. Hilary drove, Mum was in the front passenger seat, and I lent forward between the front seats to play catch.

Hilary decided to try a different driving style to mine: she drove like a complete idiot. And it worked. She was swerving erratically, accelerating hard, breaking harder, and we took corners with a dramatic squeal of tyre rubber. It was like a B-movie car chase. We were tossed about the car like ragdolls

– and it worked a treat, Mum never so much as hiccupped while Hilary was driving like this. But inevitably we reached the traffic lights and slowed into sluggish traffic – and then Mum began to heave for a hurl. And this was our thirty-minute journey to and from the hospital for each appointment: a succession of safe dangerous driving, and dangerous safe driving; as soon as the car slowed, up popped the vomit.

I went through Mum's X-ray folder at the hospital to see the initial break. It was a nasty one: the bones had snapped just above the wrist, and pushed up the arm a little. Normally this break is reset accurately with an minor operation, however the orthopaedic surgeon repositioned the bones it as best he could, (and correctly assuming that Mum's days of tennis, boxing, and mud-wrestling were over) he recommended that we agree to let the bone mend slightly out of kilter to avoid putting Mum through an unnecessary operation.

By our final visit to the hospital, for the removal of Mum's cast on **18th August**, we had our first vomit-free journey there and back again. Janet had given Mum the maximum recommended dose of anti-sickness medication; I was all plastic bags, towels and baby-wipes at the ready; and Hilary gave us another joyride of our lives. Experts, (now I know why ambulances are driven like that).

Mum continued to exist with occasional moments of brightness. She loved her food, but visiting her was sometimes a bit like visiting a mannequin, and it could take a lot of coaxing to get a response from her. Paul flew in and visited Mum in **October 2008**. He was shocked by the change in her since his previous visit when Mum was at the care home. And yet, if Mum was surprised by a jovial welcome, she could respond immediately with a great smile and a, "Och, hello darling....." (sometimes she even greeted Hilary by name; but my name had been forgotten). It just seemed to depend on the moment, it was impossible to predict a response from her.

Janet had been weaning Mum off the anti-psychotic drug that had originally been prescribed in the care home to calm her. With the doctor's approval, Janet had been reducing Mum's dosage in 2.5ml increments each month, and at this rate Mum would be completely off this drug by March 2009. It was difficult to notice an affect to this reduction in her medication, but it had to be having an affect on her quality of life, *somehow*. Paul visited again in **December 2008**, and again he was very distressed by Mum's non-responsiveness with him.

11th February 2009, Mum fell out of bed and knocked against the nightstand. No broken bones this time, but her face looked like she'd been hit with a shovel. There wasn't a lot we could do, other than move the furniture about a little to allow her an uninterrupted fall to the floor if there was to be a next time. There were siderails on her bed, but we agreed that it wouldn't be a good idea to use these, because if Mum managed to get herself over the rails she'd just have that bit further to fall.

Something that really upset me was the way Mum would grind away at her front teeth. She had been doing this for a few weeks before we noticed that her lower front teeth were half the size they should've been. Apart from that, Mum's mood was improving remarkably, and I can only suppose that this mood change may have been something to do with the fact that Janet had finally completed weaning Mum off the anti-psychotic drug.

In **late February 2009** Janet moved to a larger private nursing home in Newtownards. I was uncomfortable about this. I liked the fact that as Nursing Manager, Janet had been there for Mum to guarantee her best possible care. Janet's replacement was nice enough, but she wasn't Janet.

Over the following weeks Hilary and I became less and less impressed with Mum's care: her clothes were often left on her after they'd been soiled with spilt food and drink; she was left alone for long periods in an unlit crypt-quiet sitting room; and the new manager introduced an earlier bedtime of 6:30 every evening (with the likelihood that Mum may have been hungry again before breakfast). I completely accept that old, helpless people are a commodity; I accept that as a business, care- and nursing-homes can only increase their profits by cutting their costs here and there to make savings on their overheads; and it seemed to me that this was what was happening, at my mum's expense.

I explained to Janet how much it would mean to the family if Mum could follow her to this other private nursing home; and again, Janet very obligingly allowed Mum to jump the waiting list.

3rd April 2009, a room became available in Janet's new nursing home.

I phoned to give two-hour's notice of Mum's departure. They weren't happy – we were supposed to give four week's notice. Regardless, we bundled Mum into Hilary's car, and all her belongings in my car, and sped off to Janet's. The nursing home sent me a bill for the four-week notice period. I wrote back stating that we'd been unhappy about Mum's care since Janet had left, and that under these circumstances I wasn't going to pay for any notice period. I never heard from them again, (so either they have a rubbish solicitor, or they recognised that their quality of care *had* deteriorated since Janet had left), (four weeks nursing home care is a lot of money to forfeit).

Mum was again under the care of my sister-in-law, Janet. The differences between this, and the previous nursing home were remarkable: it was noisy with banter and laughter, there was music playing, there was hustle and bustle. And all the carers were local, all the carers demonstrated affection towards Mum, and Mum responded in kind. In the mornings Mum would often be given a big hug and a kiss by her carers to welcome her to a new day, and she was given more hugs and shows of genuine affection throughout the day by the staff. And Mum responded with huge smiles that exposed her gruesome graveyard of broken and ground teeth.

Mum began to surprise everyone with her more frequent, more enthusiastic and lucid spoken replies – something we hadn't heard for many, many months. One of the carers jokingly asked Mum if she would be putting a bet on a horse at the Aintree races on Saturday, to which Mum unexpectedly amazed everyone with, "Indeed I will <u>not</u>."

The general improvement in Mum's alertness was unbelievable. She was now sitting up in her seat, leafing through magazines with interest, answering questions in context, and really responding to her new, more tactile, more loving environment.

But she was still grinding her teeth, (it was a horrible sound, like chalk on a blackboard).

Before Mum's relocation, Janet's replacement nursing manager in the previous nursing home had told me that a dentist had examined Mum's mouth, and had prescribed medication. However, when I phoned to press her for more information she explained that she'd phoned their dentist but he had neither visited nor examined Mum's teeth, and she told me that the prescription was for one Paracetamol tablet four times a day, "Just in case." *In case of what?* In case I ask if she's being treated?

I phoned and spoke to *Mum's* dentist, and he readily agreed to give her an examination at the nursing home. In his professional opinion, if Mum wasn't suffering pain from her tooth-grinding, she ought to be; and she was also at increased risk of developing abscesses. He recommended that at least seven of Mum's teeth were removed. I agreed to have Mum referred for treatment at the hospital.

18th May 2009, I received a call from the hospital asking me to bring Mum to the dental department, first thing next morning. I arranged for a wheelchair-taxi to collect Mum and me for the return journey, and set off prepared for a long day, albeit just a preliminary examination.

As expected, Mum refused to open her mouth for the dentist; and she refused to close her mouth for an X-ray. But we finally completed the assessment, and I was told that Mum would be admitted that Thursday for an operation on Friday morning. I was nervous. They had agreed to my request to remove ALL of Mum's teeth, (to be sure she never suffered any further dental problems).

The full removal of Mum's teeth was a dramatic treatment, but it had a dramatic affect on her demeanour, (and she no longer suffered from that bad breath, the *breath of death* that had followed her since she started living at the care home in 2003).

Mum's condition over the following months remained stable, nothing remarkable seemed to happen: some days she would be in great spirits, all smiles and mumbling this and that; other days she was too sleepy to respond much. I knew from Janet that Mum *had* her moments, and I'd be told of things Mum had done or said, or responded to. Birthdays at the nursing home were celebrated with a noisy chorus of *Happy Birthday*, and there were Easter, and Halloween, and Christmas parties when the staff came to work dressed up in silly costumes, and sang songs and played games with the residents; Mum loved all this, and she would be on the edge of her seat, leaning forward, participating as much as she was able.

STAGE 6 *with Hindsight*

Mum changed a lot during this stage of her regression. She changed from being childishly silly and spontaneously animated, to occasionally withdrawn and vulnerable. Even though I was seeing Mum regularly, this sea-change in Mum's demeanour was very difficult for us to come to terms with, especially so for Paul who could only visit once or twice a year. With hindsight I can identify November '07 as when the home began to administer a sedative to control Mum's behaviour (with the best intentions – to prevent her injuring herself from her prancing about), and they must have upped the dose until she eventually became inactive and seat-bound.

Mum began to lose weight, but there wasn't a big change in her appearance until the later phase of this stage. While she was still confidently mobile we continued to escort Mum around the shopping mall for window-shopping and elevenses, and very few people noticed anything amiss with her unless she was engaged in one-to-one conversation. Little things, like her confusion about how to get into a car, were more comical than worrying. She appeared to be happy, and I'm convinced that she *was* happy.

Her first care-home was appropriate for her condition at that time, and she integrated very happily with the other residents. I was disappointed that this care-home couldn't be completely honest about the drugs that were being used to control Mum. It took a long time to wean her from the effects of this unnecessary medication, and I know that this had had a significantly negative effect on Mum's demeanour and quality of life.

For the care of both Mum and Dad, I have experienced eight care institutions. I am not a medical expert, but I qualify myself as *experienced* when it comes to care- and nursing-homes. I know how frustrating it is to be reassured that everything is "Okay", when your instincts scream otherwise. And I know how impotent I felt when I realised that Mum was being treated more as a commodity than as a human being; this must be one of the most stressful and helpless factors in trusting the care of your loved ones to others.

The correct completion of Mum's financial and legal affairs was vital, (although it was accomplished much later than I was comfortable with). The financial planning was a bit of a nightmare because Dad had left things unorganised, and the way things are with financial institutions everything was very slow to locate and liquidate and consolidate.

Everyone knows that planning for our future is important, and yet most of us put it off, indefinitely. This just means that someone else has to do it for you. Little simple things like: nominating your Power of Attorney; checking that your will is up to date and tax effective; making known the location of important documents, and so on. When someone else does this for you, you become a business to them, a bother and a frustration.

Mum's brother was disabled as a child, and he knew that old age would mean increased immobility and total dependency – and he feared this. He had already nominated Hilary and me with joint Power of Attorney for him, and when he took ill in 2005 he asked me to arrange a couple of things for him: a Living Will, that would allow him to die naturally without medical intervention or artificial resuscitation; and to arrange the donation of his body to Queen's University for medical research. I fulfilled both these requests for him, and I'm not going to pretend that it was a nice thing to do for someone I loved so much, but what he was doing was prudent planning. All his financial affairs were relatively simple to wind up after his death, and his will was up to date. Compared to the years, and years that Dad and Mum's affairs took me to complete, Mum's brother demonstrated wisdom and foresight that we should all aspire to. So, if you're thinking about sorting things out: please stop thinking about it – just do it.

Mum had a couple of bad falls during this stage of her regression. She smashed her face a couple of times, and she broke an arm. She also endured an abscess, and later began to grind away at her teeth. This sounds horrific, however, Mum never demonstrated any signs of discomfort. She had become insensitive to, or unaware of pain.

Having such a valuable and close contact in the private nursing profession has been a privilege that I have openly exploited, but it isn't something that I have ever taken for granted. Janet's timely intervention has been such a significant benefit to Mum's welfare, I really don't like to think of what conditions Mum would have suffered without her excellent management.

I realise that this insider privilege may not be available to you, and you maybe think that I've been unethical to pull strings – but *I* know that you'd do the same if you could. We are all desperate; we are all vulnerable to the established system of care for the elderly. My only other option (had it not been for Janet) would have been to plan well ahead, _well_ ahead for Mum's moving on, because waiting lists for good nursing homes are long and much sought-after.

STAGE SEVEN.

Very Severe Cognitive Decline (Severe Dementia)

All verbal abilities are lost over the course of this stage. Frequently there is no speech at all -only unintelligible utterances and rare emergence of seemingly forgotten words and phrases. Incontinent of urine, requires assistance toileting and feeding.

Basic psychomotor skills, e.g., ability to walk, are lost with the progression of this stage. The brain appears to no longer be able to tell the body what to do. Generalized rigidity and developmental neurologic reflexes are frequently present.

Global Deterioration Scale © Barry Reisberg, MD

STAGE 7 TIMELINE **March 2010 – October 2011**

Behaviour timeline:

* Noticeable decline in Mum's attentiveness.
* Rarer sporadic moments of lucidity.
* Mum entering final stage of Alzheimer's disease.
* Mum's limbs become fixed and inflexible.
* Total lack of responsiveness.

Event timeline:

* Signing the DNR order.
* Realisation that Mum was in the final stages of her condition.
* Difficulty visiting Mum while she suffers this non-responsive condition.
* Preparing for Mum's death.

By **March 2010** a change had become apparent in Mum. I couldn't put my finger on what it was exactly, but her responsiveness and wakefulness and alertness had noticeably diminished, and she was less able to remain focussed on her visitors. She was perhaps just duller.

I had been treating her with Polo Mints or Maltesers since her teeth had been removed, and she loved these. She loved these sweets so much that, as soon as she heard my voice, Mum would now greet me with her outstretched tongue, eager to accept the sweet stimulation and full flavour. This became a bit of a joke, as every time I'd speak to her she'd stick her tongue out; and when I leaned in to kiss her hello or goodbye I'd be met with this wanting tongue again, (not what a son wants from his mum).

Yet despite Mum's continued mental regression, she'd surprise us with a less occasional toothless mumble, such as "Och, hello darling," or "Hello honey-bunny." And Janet told me that on one occasion one of the other residents had caused a disturbance in the lounge, and the atmosphere was very tense while the carers tried to calm the situation, and Mum broke the silence, declaring "You're just an ignoramus." And everyone burst out laughing.

Mum became typically inactive and unresponsive, but she could still waken out of this condition with beaming smiles and the occasional mumbled affection.

5th May 2010 Hilary and I signed a *Do Not Resuscitate Order* (DNR) for Mum. This had been on our to-do list for a long time, but despite the fact that we wanted this for Mum, signing it wasn't easy.

The main reason for signing the DNR order was because Mum's naturally weakened condition had made her more susceptible to common diseases. The last thing we wanted for Mum was a doctor instructing that she be removed to hospital. This sounds terrible, but the distress this would cause Mum, (in our opinion, and in the professional opinion of the nursing staff at the nursing home), being removed to a hospital, and possibly an attempt to resuscitate being made on her frail body – it simply wasn't appropriate. Signing the DNR didn't mean that we didn't love Mum; it meant that we love her enough to allow her to die with some dignity in the care of people who know her. If Mum became ill, she would be treated within the nursing home, but she would only be offered non-aggressive palliative care. As a Christian, I knew that Mum had no fear of death; as a Human Being I knew that Mum may still have a natural fear of dying. Signing this order wasn't something Hilary or I (having joint Power of Attorney for Mum) did without very careful consideration (more than a year of very careful consideration).

Paul flew in for another visit with Mum on 13th November 2010. We'd anticipated a difficult meeting for Paul, much like the non-responsive ones he'd enjoyed before – only worse. Hilary and I agreed to meet him at the nursing home to try and make his visit less of a shocking non-event for him. I arrived first and gave Mum her breakfast, then wheeled her round to meet Paul at the front door.

Mum muttered a little and gave Paul a couple of big smiles and knowing nods (as if she remembered him). But when I pulled out her little piano keyboard to play a couple of the tunes that Mum used to play at home (Beethoven, and Chopin, and Joplin) Paul was really affected. I think for the first time in several years he saw that Mum is still *in there* somewhere somehow, (and the music brought back so many memories for him). He could clearly see that Mum wasn't *always* vacant (as she had been on most of his previous visits).

By **mid-May 2011** neither Hilary nor I had managed to persuade much of a response from Mum for perhaps six or seven weeks. She would automatically respond to a mint by sticking her tongue out to accept it, but this was performed with her eyes closed and with no other signs of mental activity.

With a lot of effort we could sometime raise a little smile, but generally Mum existed in a state of stupid non-responsiveness.

I asked Janet what the next stage of Alzheimer's disease would be for Mum; she hesitantly replied, "There *isn't* a next stage." This was the final stage.

Mum still enjoyed her mealtimes, and she slept soundly at night. The rest of the time she was on constant flat battery mode with little interest in anything, apparently. And yet, very rarely, she might open her eyes, smile, and mumble a greeting before returning to her unconsciousness (but it was pure chance whether Hilary or I were there to witness this).

Mum's arms and legs had become fixed into a seated position from which we couldn't un-bend her. But why would we *want* to un-bend her, she wasn't going anywhere.

I contacted the few friends and relations whom I knew still tried to make time to visit Mum, to explain that they needn't feel bad if they didn't visit anymore, because it was unlikely that Mum would even recognise the fact that they were with her. I knew that her friends felt that they *should* visit, and I did feel wick explaining this to them – but Mum was now oblivious to visitors (including me), and unless they felt a strong duty of love to visit, they shouldn't suffer the needless distress. Mum was only really responding to being lifted by the nursing staff – even her eating had become robotic.

Visiting Mum became very difficult and distressing for Hilary and me; seeing her in such a state of nothingness, without the ability to respond, unconscious to the world, it has been *extremely* disheartening.

In **June 2011** I made Mum a coffin. It sounds awful because she wasn't dead, but I'd just made one at the request of a close friend who was dying; and understanding what it had meant to my dying friend, I realised that Mum would have wanted the same. I made it from a beech tree felled in Tullymore Forest at the foot of the Mourne Mountains; made without nails or screws, and finished with a single coat of hand-rubbed wax. And I dreaded having to use it, (and yes, it *is* kind of embarrassing admitting to having a coffin ready for my mum). I'm not ready for Mum to die. I'm more prepared for her death than I was with Dad's, or Mum's brother; I've had years and years to prepare for Mum's ultimate appointment, but it doesn't make it any easier to think about.

STAGE 7 *with Hindsight*

This has been the most heartbreaking stage of Mum's condition since she was first diagnosed. It's like we're just waiting for her to die, (which I *am*, I suppose, because there isn't a *next* stage).

Obviously, visiting someone is easier when it's a two-way conversation, even if the other person can't speak, seeing that they are responding positively to your *being there* is rewarding. But to visit someone as close to you as your own mum, and to have no response, no reaction, no nothing, it's just soul-destroying.

Mum is immobile (actually, she is fixed in a sort of foetal position in the shape of her seat) and she must be handled with care by two experienced carers. Her only movement appears to be her ability to eat and swallow, although even her swallow fails occasionally. Janet tells me that most patients with Mum's advanced stage of Alzheimer's disease are bedbound, but because Mum's heart is still strong she is able to sit in her recliner and achieve *some* stimulation from the comings and goings around her, (for now, anyhow).

Visiting Mum is not a pleasure anymore: it's a duty. It's often traumatising, always depressing. Soul destroying. I wonder if she realises her existence, if she is aware of *anything*.

I have been first on the scene of a bad car crash a couple of times, and in each case the cars were destroyed, but the radio was still chirpily singing away to the injured passengers. In a way this reminds me of Mum; in a way she is trapped within a useless body, but her little radio refuses to quit; it is only the dwindling strength of Mum's heartbeat that keeps her alive, everything else has given up.

THE END....

Mum isn't dead. (When I was with her this afternoon she was doing a pretty good impression of being dead, but her heart is still quietly pulsing.) Mum is in the last phase of the final stage of Alzheimer's disease. She is alive, but she isn't living; she is barely existing. By the time you read this it's very likely that Mum *will* be dead. However, as I write this, although Mum's life and suffering with Alzheimer's disease hasn't concluded, my story ends.

Everyone's circumstances are different.

I've not written this account of Mum's disease and care as a *How To....* And I'm certainly not looking for sympathy. My primary motive has been to illustrate the disease, and its effects on the sufferer and the family. My main motive has been to allow you to recognise the many mistakes that I have made in the care for my Mum, in the hope that you'll avoid repeating them.

I realise that Mum's diagnosis was late; her stress from caring for Dad clouded many warning signals that should have alerted us years earlier to a potential mental health problem. I know that when Alzheimer's is recognised early there are now new and more effective drugs that can slow the disease and allow the sufferer to live a relatively normal life.

However, despite her late diagnosis, with hindsight I can still appreciate how well things worked out for Mum's care. It could've been much worse.

I recently heard a news report of a man who had cared for his wife who was suffering advanced Alzheimer's. He suffocated his wife rather than watch her suffer further decline. I can fully understand his distress. I can fully understand his motives. And I fully sympathise with him. Whether he made the correct decision isn't something I would ever judge, that's between him and God; but I know that his action was not only a deed born of desperation, his was a deed born of love and respect.

It's easy to ask myself, "Why Mum?" Why such a beautiful, shining, loving human being? She didn't deserve to have her life robbed by such a disease. It's easy to question divine wisdom like this, but what I *should* declare is that *without* divine involvement this *would* have been a much worse experience:

Without the option of Hilary's career break to care for Mum at home for a full year; without the flexibility of my self-employment that allowed me to spend so much time sorting things correctly for Mum; and without the timely intervention of my well-placed sister-in-law, this <u>*would*</u> have been a very different story, (a tragic story of helplessness, much greater stress, and much, much more unhappiness), (which may have led to *my* conviction for euthanasia).

For all of the beneficial factors that have contributed to Mum's care I cannot accept the concept of either luck, or coincidence. I can only accept that through Mum's faith and our prayers, God has been the main carer in Mum's life. With the clarity of hindsight I can now appreciate this fact, and despite the horrible unfairness of Alzheimer's disease, I can never take for granted His grace and care for each one of us.

ABOUT THE AUTHOR

Brian Bailie lives in a wee cottage in the green lumpy landscape between the lough and the sea, on the Ards Peninsula of County Down, Northern Ireland.
In his field, he is a well-known product designer and owner of an international manufacturing business based in industrial east coast China.

However, Brian is first and foremost a son. When his mother's dementia was first diagnosed his world was turned upside-down, and his business was put on hold while he attempted to provide the best care for her.

Brian's other books include: Prepare Yourself for China, the visitor's survival guide to China ; and, The Broncle, a curious tale of adoption and reunion.

www.broncle.com

12627748R00070

Made in the USA
Charleston, SC
17 May 2012